INTERMITTENT FASTING DIET

Step-by-step guide to Burn Fat, Boost Energy Lose

Weight, Get Smarter, and Live Your Longest, Healthiest Lifestyle.

BY Melissa White

SECOND EDITION
UPDATE CHAPTER 3

3

4

Chapter 1. Intermittent Fasting: A Potential Diet Plan for Successful Brain Aging

The weakness of the sensory system to propelling age is very regularly show in neurodegenerative issues like Alzheimer's and Parkinson's illnesses. In this survey article we depict proof recommending that two dietary intercessions, caloric limitation (CR) and intermittent fasting (IF), can draw out the wellbeing range of the sensory system by impinging upon major metabolic and cell flagging pathways that manage life-length. CR and IF influence energy and oxygen extremist digestion, and cell stress reaction frameworks, in manners that secure neurons against hereditary and natural components to which they would somehow or another capitulate during maturing. There are numerous intelligent pathways and sub-atomic systems by which CR and IF advantage neurons including those including insulin-like flagging, FoxO record factors, sirtuins and peroxisome proliferator-initiated receptors. These pathways invigorate the creation of protein chaperones, neurotrophic elements and cancer prevention agent chemicals, all of which help cells adapt to pressure and oppose illness. A superior comprehension of the effect of CR and IF on the maturing sensory system will probably prompt novel methodologies for forestalling and treating neurodegenerative problems.

1.1 Introduction

Mind issues of maturing have as of late become driving reasons for handicap and passing, because of various advances in the anticipation and therapy of cardiovascular sickness and tumors. A few noticeable danger factors for significant age-related illnesses, like cardiovascular sickness, type 2 diabetes and malignant growths, are likewise hazard factors for some neurodegenerative infections. These danger factors incorporate a fatty eating regimen, nutrient inadequacies (for example folic corrosive and cell reinforcements) and an inactive way of life. Examination endeavors on neurodegenerative problems have quickly extended in the previous decade and those endeavors have prompted many promising restorative intercessions to increment both wellbeing length and life expectancy. Numerous individuals live for at least eighty years and appreciate a well-working cerebrum for the duration of their life expectancy. We subsequently realize that the human mind is fit for maturing effectively. We are currently at a phase where our insight into both the hereditary and ecological elements which have been connected to fruitless cerebrum maturing, and their phone and sub-atomic results, can be used to furnish everyone with guidance on maturing effectively. In this audit, we will examine two dietary systems, caloric limitation and intermittent fasting, which might actually be utilized to intervene fruitful maturing and prevent the beginning of certain neurodegenerative issues.

Dietary limitation and the sound maturing of man. Accepting Da Vinci's Man as a paragon of mankind we have depicted how he may live past the years ordinarily attributed to renaissance Homo sapiens through modifications in caloric admission. Both gross and cell physiology is significantly influenced by caloric limitation (CR) or intermittent fasting (IF) systems. As for net physiology there is obviously a critical decrease of muscle versus fat and mass, which upholds a solid cardiovascular framework and diminishes episodes of myocardial localized necrosis. Notwithstanding cardio security a more noteworthy resilience to stretch is incited in the liver, the supplement center of Homo sapiens. The presence of elective energy stores, for example, ketone bodies (for example beta-hydroxybutyrate) empower Homo sapiens to endure extra anxieties of life. Exorbitant and pernicious blood glucose is shortened by an upgraded affectability to insulin and glucose and its usage as a fuel source. The rise of neurotropic factors likewise upholds the support of complex neuronal circuits needed for memory maintenance and discernment. At the atomic level large numbers of the valuable impacts of CR/IF are restated. Proteins and nucleic acids are shielded from harming post-translational adjustments by means of up guidelines of sirtuin histone deacetylases and heat stun proteins (Hsp). To keep up Man during the useful times of fasting, peroxisome proliferator-actuated receptors (PPAR) are enacted to prepare fat stores for energy utilization. During these seasons of energy shortage, cell endurance is upheld by the enactment of fork head box-other (FoxO) record factors and through the age of neurotropic specialists, for example, mind determined neurotropic factor (BDNF). Incendiary cytokines, up controlled by CR/IF can even serve to permit improved synaptic strength during the hours of energy shortage.

1.2 Actions of Molecules Involved in Aging and Degeneration

An expanding number of hereditary and ecological variables are being distinguished that can deliver neurons helpless against the maturing cycle. A comprehension of how such causal or inclining hazard factors advance neuronal brokenness as well as death is basic for creating ways to deal with save useful neuronal circuits. Likewise, to other organ frameworks, cells in the mind experience a combined weight of oxidative and metabolic pressure that might be a widespread element of the maturing cycle. Expanded oxidative pressure during cerebrum maturing can be found in every one of the significant classes of cell particles, including proteins, lipids and nucleic acids. Some oxidative changes of proteins that have been seen in neurons during maturing incorporate carbonyl development, covalent adjustments of cysteine, and lysine and histidine deposits by the lipid peroxidation item 4-hydroxynonenal, nitration of proteins on tyrosine buildups, and glycation. A typical oxidative change of DNA, seen during mind maturing is the arrangement of 8-hydroxydeoxyguanosine. Every one of these changes of proteins, lipids and nucleic acids are additionally exacerbated in various degenerative problems like Alzheimer's infection (AD) and Parkinson's sickness (PD). Advertisement can be brought about by changes in the qualities encoding the amyloid forerunner protein (APP) as well as presenilin-1 (PS-1) or - 2 (PS-

2). Every one of these changes brings about an expanded creation of amyloid-beta peptide which itself can build the oxidative weight on neurons. Advertisement prompts a reformist disintegration of psychological capacity with a deficiency of memory. Neuronal injury is consequently present in locales of the cerebrum that include the hippocampus and the cortex. Advertisement is portrayed by two principle obsessive trademarks that comprise of extracellular plaques of amyloid-beta peptide totals, and intracellular neurofibrillary tangles made out of the hyperphosphorylated microtubule-related protein tau. The beta-amyloid statement that comprises the plaques is made out of a 39–42 amino corrosive peptide, which is the proteolytic result of the APP protein. Curiously, the APP and presenilin changes have likewise been appeared to diminish levels of a discharged type of APP that has been appeared to advance synaptic pliancy (learning and memory) and endurance of neurons. PD is likewise a moderately regular reformist neurodegenerative issue influencing around 1% of the populace more seasoned than the age of 65 years and roughly 4–5% of the populace more established than the age of 85. It is brought about by a particular degeneration of the dopamine neurons in the substantia nigra. PD is portrayed by quake, unbending nature and gradualness of developments. Non-engine highlights, like dementia and dysautonomia, happen regularly, particularly in the high level phases of the sickness.

1.3 Health-Span and Life-Span Extension by Intermittent Fasting

Since forever, various social orders have perceived the advantageous consequences for wellbeing and general prosperity of restricting food consumption for specific timeframes, either for strict reasons or when food was scant. The principal generally perceived logical investigation of limited eating regimens and their capacity to expand life-range was distributed. It showed that taking care of subjects with an eating regimen containing inedible cellulose drastically broadened both mean and most extreme life expectancy in these creatures. Numerous investigations have affirmed this outcome and stretched out it to subject and different species including organic product flies nematodes, water bugs, arachnids and fish.

In this audit we will endeavor to demonstrate how, with dietary change, not exclusively life-length can be broadened yet in addition conceivably, wellbeing range, for example a great time wherein we have an illness/pathology free mien. We will likewise research through which sub-atomic components the advantages, in general living being, of dietary admission alteration are inferred. Varieties of this essential dietary system, presently known as caloric limitation (CR), are the best method of expanding the life expectancy of warm blooded animals without hereditarily adjusting them. All the more as of late, another variety of CR, intermittent fasting (IF) or each and every other day taking care of (EODF), has additionally been appeared to expand life-length and have advantageous wellbeing impacts. Subjects kept up on calorie-confined eating regimens are for the most part more modest and more slender and have less muscle versus fat and more modest significant organs than not indispensable took care of creatures. They are by and large more dynamic, which may identify with the need to look for food, and the typical age-related abatement in actual work is extraordinarily decreased in calorie-limited creatures. In any case, these creatures are more helpless against cold temperatures, which is a significant wellspring of mortality for little warm blooded animals (Berry and Bronson, 1992). The sum by which life-length is stretched out has been appeared to increment continuously as caloric admission is diminished, until the place of starvation. The hour of beginning of the dietary limitation (for example pre-or post-pubertal) and the term of the CR system additionally decide the sum by which life-range is broadened. Vitally both CR and IF can decrease the seriousness of hazard factors for sicknesses like diabetes and cardiovascular infection in subjects. In numerous examinations, execution of the IF dietary system brings about an around 20–30% decrease in caloric admission over the long haul. Upkeep of rats on this other day CR taking care of routine for 2–4 months brings about obstruction of hippocampal neurons to synthetically induced. In a water maze spatial learning task, this decreased damage to hippocampal neurons is also linked to a striking preservation of learning and memory. As a result, these dietary regimens may be beneficial for crippling and common neurodegenerative disorders like Alzheimer's, Huntington's, and Parkinson's disease.

Information from the creature considers depicted in this audit show that neurons in the cerebrums of subjects and subject kept up on CR or IF regimens display expanded protection from oxidative, metabolic and excitotoxic affronts. The basic inquiry to pose regarding these examinations is, what are the hidden atomic components that represent the insurance against this heap of intense cell affronts? Examiners have tended to this significant inquiry by estimating various proteins and lipids that are known to assume a part in ensuring neurons against a wide range of affronts. We will examine and exhibit what a complex physiological reaction to CR/IF happens in the living being and how this may in the long run mean sound maturing.

Responses of Stress

From nature we realize that the securing of accessible food structures quite possibly the most significant conduct sets and subsequently evacuation of sufficient food sources goes about as an extraordinary main thrust for engrained conduct and causes a specific level of mental and physiological pressure in the organic entity. This worldview, as with such countless parts of science, stretches out even to the basic physiological and cell measures inside the creature. To epitomize this, few distinctive pressure proteins have been estimated in the minds from subjects kept up on either not obligatory or CR eats less for a very long time. Instances of such pressure proteins incorporate warmth stun proteins and glucose-managed proteins. These atomic chaperone proteins associate with a wide range of proteins in cells and capacity to guarantee their legitimate collapsing, from one perspective, and corruption of harmed proteins, then again. They may likewise interface with, and adjust the capacity of, apoptotic proteins including caspases. Levels of a portion of these chaperone proteins might be expanded during the maturing interaction as a defensive reaction. Cell culture and in vivo examines have shown that heat-stun protein-70 (HSP-70) and glucose-controlled protein 78 (GRP-78) can secure neurons against injury and demise in trial models of neurodegenerative issues. Levels of HSP-70 and GRP-78 were discovered to be expanded in the cortical, hippocampal and striatal neurons of the CR subjects contrasted with the age-coordinated with not indispensable took care of creatures. Past examinations in this and different research centers have given proof that HSP-70 and GRP-78 can ensure neurons against excitotoxic and oxidative injury, which recommends that they add to the neuroprotective impact of CR. This information may exhibit that CR can prompt a gentle pressure reaction in neurons, probably because of a diminished energy, fundamentally glucose, accessibility. Notwithstanding these subcellular stress reactions, it has been accounted for that IF brings about expanded degrees of coursing corticosterone, which is typically related decidedly with the pressure condition of the creature. As opposed to impeding stressors, like constant wild pressure, which jeopardize neurons through glucocorticoid receptor actuation, intermittent fasting IF down directs glucocorticoid receptors with upkeep of mineralocorticoid receptors in neurons which can act to forestall neuronal harm and passing. It is possible that exchanging times of anabolism and catabolism, happening during IF, may assume an unthinking part in setting off expansions in cell stress obstruction and the maintenance of harmed proteins and cells.

Inordinate neurological pressure regularly appears as raised degrees of glutamatergic neurotransmission, for example in post ischemic occasions or epileptic seizures there can be an over-burden of cells with calcium, incited by the plain glutamate discharge that outcomes in possible cell passing. This type of excitoxic cell passing can be mirrored by the infusion of kainic corrosive (KA) into the cerebral ventricles/cerebrum areas of exploratory creatures. When the excitotoxic KA is infused into the dorsal hippocampus of subject it instigates seizures and harm to pyramidal neurons in areas CA3 and CA1. A critical expansion in the endurance of CA3 and CA1 neurons in the IF subject contrasted and subject took care of not indispensable, after the kainic affront has been illustrated.

Neurotropic Factors

As both IF and CR prompt a gentle pressure reaction in synapses this can bring about the initiation of repaying instruments, for example the up guideline of neurotropic factors, for example, BDNF and glial cell line-inferred neurotropic factor (GDNF) just as the previously mentioned heat stun proteins. On the off chance that regimens have been shown to enhance and lessen neuronal harm and improve the useful result in creature models of neurological injury, for example, stroke and furthermore neurodegenerative issues like Parkinson's infection, and Huntington's illness. The neuroprotective component of IF isn't known, yet it has been accounted for that IF prompts the creation of cerebrum determined neurotropic factor (BDNF) which was related with expanded hippocampal neurogenesis in subjects and subject. One of the essential neuroprotective systems ascribed to BDNF gives off an impression of being the capacity of BDNF-intervened enactment of its related TrkB receptor which at that point entrains incitement of numerous flagging pathways. Noticeable among these TrkB flagging pathways is the phosphatidyl inositol 3-kinase (PI3K)/protein kinase B (Akt) pathway that has been embroiled in a few of the CR/IF defensive components that will be examined at more noteworthy length in this audit.

Ketone bodies

Dietary fasting is known to bring about an expanded creation of ketone bodies, for example beta-hydroxybutyrate, which can be utilized by the creature as a fuel source notwithstanding restricted glucose accessibility. Regarding ketogenesis apparently IF regimens appear to be more agreeable to this energy creation pathway than more exacting CR conventions. Subject on IF regimens have been appeared to burden normal more than subject on CR regimens. They likewise have bigger fat stores and a more prominent ketogenic reaction than CR subject. On the off chance that dietary systems can build up a two-overlay expansion in the fasting serum centralization of beta-hydroxybutyrate contrasted and subject took care of not indispensable. This shift to ketogenesis may assume an immediate part in the cytoprotective impacts of IF, in light of the fact that it has been accounted for that subjects took care of a ketogenic diet show expanded protection from seizures, and that beta-hydroxybutyrate itself can ensure neurons in subjects of Alzheimer's and Parkinson's infections. Ketogenic counts calories, which advance a metabolic shift from glucose usage to ketogenesis, are additionally recommended for certain patients with epilepsy as this is prophylactic against the reformist excitotoxic neuronal harm and debasement that can happen if the condition is untreated.

Glucose and Insulin Signaling

During fasting or dietary limitation the essential adjustment to the creature is the accessibility of glucose for oxidative breath. The systems by which energy is gotten from substitute sources or how the leftover glucose is taken care of are fitting to the extrapolation of the medical advantages of CR/IF regimens. The significance of glucose taking care of proficiency for sound maturing can be exhibited by the way that glucose levels in the blood, incorporated over the long haul, have been proposed to prompt undeniable degrees of non-enzymatic glycation, a type of protein harm. CR has been appeared to explicitly constrict oxyradical creation and harm and non-enzymatic glycation.

Both IF and CR regimens effectsly affect insulin and glucose levels, for example decrease, yet curiously they effectsly affect serum IGF-1 levels and serum beta-hydroxybutyrate levels, for example both these boundaries are expanded with intermittent fasting IF contrasted with CR. A longitudinal report on male subjects exhibited that CR diminished the mean 24-h plasma glucose focus by around 15 mg/dl and the insulin fixation by about half. CR system creatures used glucose at similar rate as did the subjects took care of not indispensable, notwithstanding the lower plasma glucose and especially lower plasma insulin levels. Hence, it is suggested that CR either expands glucose adequacy or insulin responsiveness or both, and that the support of low degrees of glucose and insulin control the useful and life-broadening activities of CR. CR has likewise been found to lessen plasma glucose and insulin fixations in fasting rhesus monkeys. Furthermore, CR can build insulin affectability in rhesus and cynomolgus monkeys. A significant justification this accentuation being set on the insulin–glucose control framework in maturing is the finding that deficiency of-work changes of the insulin flagging framework bring about existence augmentation in three species: C. elegans, D. melanogaster, and subject. Generally, from numerous test studies, CR and IF appear to persistently lessen the flowing degrees of insulin bringing about an inevitable improved glucose preparation and an upgraded insulin affectability, the two of which serve to keep a stockpile of glucose for the essential organs, focal sensory system and balls to help these basic organs on schedule of restricted energy admission. The genuine decrease of insulin receptor flagging interceded by diminished plasma insulin levels has an effect additionally on a few different elements that significantly sway upon the cell reaction to CR/IF; this will be examined in later segments.

Cytokines

There is mounting proof to recommend that provocative cycles could be fundamentally associated with the improvement old enough related pathologies, for example, those saw in Alzheimer's sickness. The enactment of microglia in light of injury or during maturing causes the acceptance of a fiery like reaction. This reaction is exemplified and started by an improved articulation of interleukin-1 in the animated microglia. Considering this it is hence obvious that fiery cytokines may likewise be ensnared in the CR/IF-interceded measures that improve this neurodegeneration. Late discoveries recommend that IFN is a significant go between of neuronal pliancy, for example IFN may improve synaptogenesis, direct synaptic pliancy and control neurogenesis.

It was as of late revealed that degrees of IFN are expanded in flowing leukocytes of monkeys that had been kept up on a CR diet. It has additionally been shown that CR lifts the statement of IFN in the hippocampus where it applies an excitoprotective activity of IFN. Cytokines can likewise be delivered by instinctive organs outside the insusceptible framework and the focal sensory system. Fat tissue, which amasses during maturing and is explicitly diminished upon CR or IF regimens, can go about as an endocrine organ, which produces trophic chemicals that are dynamic all through the body, for example tumor putrefaction factor (TNF). TNF has additionally been appeared to trigger insulin opposition in creatures. In vitro cell-culture examines have shown that TNF renders cells insulin safe through a down guideline of glucose carrier union just as through obstruction with insulin receptor flagging pathways which we have seen are fundamentally engaged with sound maturing. In vivo, the shortfall of the TNF receptor essentially improves insulin affectability which copies the insulin-related impacts found in CR/IF creatures. Curiously, it has been shown that CR constricts the age-related up guideline of atomic factor (NF), which is a record factor that initiates the statement of TNF in fat tissue and the creation of fiery cytokines in resistant cells. In this way constriction of TNF instigated insulin obstruction may upgrade the glucose use limit of the organic entity, subsequently fighting off the unfavorable impacts of exorbitant blood glucose that may happen in the midst of chronic weakness and with propelling age.

Adipose and Satiety-Generated hormones

Leptin and adiponectin are two chemicals that are normally connected with the input control of hunger and satiety. Both of these variables are created by fat tissue which is obviously significantly influenced by CR/IF systems. Notwithstanding its job in satiety, leptin, delivered into the dissemination, diminishes the degree of stress chemicals and builds thyroid action and thyroid-chemical levels which both outcome in expanded energy use. As we have seen, CR regimens will in general up manage pressure chemicals in an okay way and moreover they can down control thyroid chemicals, possibly through this constriction of flowing leptin levels. Anyway leptin's part in interceding the valuable impacts of CR might be optional to its satiety job as it has been shown that subject that need leptin lamentably exhibit a decreased life expectancy, contrasted with not obligatory creatures, and are corpulent. Adiponectin has been appeared to trigger expanded insulin affectability by means of up guideline of AMP-initiated protein kinase. This kinase directs glucose and fat digestion in muscle in light of energy limit, and has been appeared to secure neurons against metabolic pressure. Significantly, adiponectin levels ascend during CR, which recommends that this fat determined chemical may likewise have a significant contributory job in the physiological shift to an upgraded insulin affectability in these creatures. Late discoveries show that subject that have been hereditarily designed to be lean live more. Surely, tissue-explicit knockout of the insulin receptor in fat cells keeps the tissue from putting away fat, which brings about lean creatures that live altogether more than wild-type subject. These information propose that instinctive fat may be particularly significant in driving insulin obstruction and pathogenesis.

Sirtuins

As lower life forms, for example yeast and nematode worms, have an impressively more limited life expectancy than well evolved creatures they have demonstrated valuable for the revelation of the atomic determinants of sound life span. It has gotten evident that among the different variables that have been recognized that control life-range in these lower organic entities, a considerable lot of these additionally interface the change of caloric admission to the expansion in wellbeing length so wanted by dietary mediations of sickness measures.

One of the essential hereditary determinants of replicative life expectancy to rise out of hereditary examinations in yeast is the quiet data controller 2 (SIR2). The SIR2 quality was meant on the grounds that it intercedes a particular quality hushing activity. Inhibitory changes of SIR2 can abbreviate life-range, and expanded quality measurements of SIR2 broadened life-length. The SIR2 ortholog in C. elegans was correspondingly demonstrated to be a vital determinant of the life expectancy around there. As yeast and C. elegans separated from a typical precursor around one billion years prior this may propose that relatives of that predecessor, including warm blooded animals, will have SIR2-related qualities engaged with controlling their life expectancy. As dietary guideline has additionally demonstrated to be an amazing modulator of life expectancy it is sensible to guess that CR/IF and SIR2 qualities may join to assume a significant part in these numerous and complex physiological pathways. Mammalian homologues of the yeast SIR2 quality have in this way been found and strangely the SIR2 ortholog, SIRT1, may to a limited extent intervene an expansive cluster of physiological impacts that happen in creatures on a changed eating routine, beit CR or IF. The group of proteins found that are encoded for by the mammalian SIR2 homologues are all in all named sirtuins. A few late reports have shown increments in SIRT1 protein levels because of food hardship. Furthermore SIR up guideline has been appeared in light of cell stressors, like high osmolarity, subsequently the sirtuin group of proteins could be effectively directed by the gentle, controllable pressure initiated by CR/IF. Sirtuins have a moderately uncommon enzymatic limit as they are NAD-subordinate histone deacetylases. The mammalian SIRT1 quality item chemical can, notwithstanding histones, deacetylate numerous different substrates. In such manner, SIRT1 was as of late appeared to deacetylate and down regulate NF. It is interesting to guess that the up guideline of SIRT1 by CR adds to the noticed expansion in insulin affectability and decrease in irritation, conceivably through the control of the NF/TNF pathways.

It have proposed an atomic pathway for SIR2 enactment that possibly interfaces modifications in caloric admission to life-range expansion. Upon CR/IF there is an underlying expansion in oxygen utilization and breath, to the detriment of fermentative cycles. Maturation is a commonplace component by which cells can create ATP and furthermore store overabundance energy as ethanol when glucose is plentiful. This metabolic shift triggers an attending decrease in NADH levels. NADH goes about as a serious inhibitor of SIR2, so its decrease during CR/IF periods would be required to up manage the compound and subsequently broaden the organic entity's life expectancy in accordance with yeast and C. elegans considers. Steady with this, removal of mitochondrial electron transport hindered the impact of CR on life-range, and overexpressing NADH dehydrogenase, the compound that shunts electrons from NADH to the electron transport chain, expanded the creature's life expectancy. Hence it shows up then that CR/IF initiates a more effective utilization of glucose by means of an increment in breath. Notwithstanding this there is a change in muscle cells from utilizing glucose, which is somewhat, processed in not indispensable creatures fermentatively (delivering lactate), at the utilization of unsaturated fats, which are oxidatively used. This shift saves glucose for the mind, forestalling neurodegeneration, and connects with the trademark upgrade of insulin affectability in muscle and liver found in CR. Albeit the activities of sirtuins in the sensory system are simply starting to be investigated, it has been accounted for that SIR2 (SIRT1 in vertebrates) actuation through expanded quality measurements or treatment with the sirtuin activator resveratrol can secure neurons against the pathogenic impacts of polyglutamine-extended huntingtin proteins in worm and mouse models of Huntington's infection.

Sirtuins likewise appear to assume a part in interceding the successful job of fat tissue in the physiological transaction of the advantages of CR/IF systems to the living being. Perhaps the main controllers of fat tissue work is the peroxisome proliferator-actuated record factor receptor gamma. This receptor goes about as an atomic record factor that controls numerous qualities associated with cell endurance and reactions to metabolic changes. One PPAR quality objective, the aP2 quality, encodes a protein that helps fat stockpiling. SIRT1 can go about as a repressor of PPAR, in this way down directing qualities, for example, the mouse aP2 quality. During fasting SIRT1 enactment is trailed by an improved restricting to the aP2 advertiser in fat tissue. This causes a restraint of aP2 quality articulation causing a possible advancement of fat assembly into the blood to help the life form's energy balance. Endless supply of caloric admission there is a traditionalist enactment of SIRT1 in fat tissue, which acts to lessen fat stores and likely resets hormonal levels to change the speed of maturing. This methodology likewise bodes well when it is viewed as that effective proliferation is additionally managed by muscle versus fat and is stopped during CR, possibly to continue when accessible energy supplies become more bountiful.

Peroxisome proliferator-activated receptor and co-factors

PPARs, as we have seen, are individuals from the atomic chemical receptor subfamily of record factors. PPARs structure useful heterodimers with retinoid X receptors (RXRs) and these heterodimers manage record of different qualities. There are three known subtypes of PPARs. These atomic receptor record factors manage qualities associated with supplement transport and digestion just as protection from stress. PPARs themselves additionally enlist different proteins notwithstanding the RXR to intercede their total capacity. One such protein is the peroxisome proliferator-actuated receptor (PPAR) co-activator 1 (PGC-1). This co-activator has been demonstrated to be firmly managed by dietary change in lower creatures and higher warm blooded animals.

PGC-1 exists in two isoforms, and these isoforms have arisen as unmistakable controllers of the versatile reactions to caloric hardship. PGC-1 manages the ligand-subordinate and - free initiation of an enormous number of atomic receptors including the PPARs. There has been accounted for an age-subordinate decrease in PGC-1 which may fuel the maturing cycle. Anyway in subject and primates CR has been appeared to invert this age-subordinate decline in PGC-1, PPAR and directed qualities

PGC-1, the main PGC relative recognized was described as a protein that associates with the PPAR to manage earthy colored fat separation during variation to cold pressure. This virus stress might be viewed as closely resembling the physiological and mental pressure instigated by caloric limitation. During CR/IF periods, when insulin levels are low, PGC-1 and PGC-1 beta quality articulation is improved in subjects. PGC-1 was likewise prompted in the livers of subject and subjects after longer term CR. PGC-1 and beta can coordinately direct qualities associated with gluconeogenesis and unsaturated fat beta-oxidation in various organs during fasting. Both these cycles are useful to the upkeep of a sound energy balance in the midst of restricted food. Thus through PPAR initiation additional provisions of glucose can be assembled and substitute fuel sources can be misused. Just as PGC guideline during fasting, PPAR is additionally up directed by fasting in liver, little and digestive organ, thymus and pancreas. Countless qualities engaged with unsaturated fat beta-oxidation, known to be directed by PPAR are likewise expanded in articulation because of fasting. During times of fasting PPAR take out subject show a powerlessness to direct qualities associated with unsaturated fat beta-and oxidation and ketogenesis in the liver, kidney and heart alongside absence of control of blood levels of glucose or ketone bodies.

Not exclusively is the liver the energy-directing center of warm blooded animals however it additionally addresses perhaps the main stores of glycogen, supplements and nutrients. One would accordingly anticipate that there would be a basic connection between adjustments of caloric admission and resultant hepatic capacity. Along these lines it has been shown that CR shields the liver from a wide scope of natural stressors, a significant number of which instigate harm through flowing fiery arbiters. PPAR has been appeared to direct hepatic reactions to different types of pressure. Subject pre-presented to PPAR agonists show diminished cell harm, expanded tissue fix, and diminished mortality after openness to various physical and synthetic hepatic stressors. Apparently utilitarian PPAR are vital for the CR-intervened assurance of the liver from harm instigated by hepatotoxicants like thioacetamide. In particular, it was shown by that PPAR take out subject, as opposed to wild-type subject, were not shielded from thioacetamide by CR systems. Lipid peroxide levels, related with oxidative cell stress in the fringe and the focal sensory system, are likewise altogether expanded in maturing. PPAR take out subject show a checked height in lipid peroxidation items contrasted with wild-type subject. Hence PPAR may impact maturing through the guideline of various harm and fix measures after openness to a plenty of endogenous or natural stressors.

PGC-1 isoforms are transcriptionally or post transnationally directed in well evolved creatures by a few flagging pathways embroiled in the association between CR/IF and life-length augmentation. These incorporate fork head box "other" (FoxO) record factors (through an insulin/insulin-like development factor-I - subordinate pathway), glucagon-invigorated cell AMP (cAMP) reaction component restricting protein (CREB), stress-enacted protein kinases (p38 and N-terminal kinase) and obviously SIRT1. We will talk about next how these elements connect to control the atomic instruments of CR/IF that sway upon interpretation to sound maturing.

Transcription Factors of FoxO

In warm blooded animals, insulin and IGF-I tie to one or the other insulin or IGF-1 receptors initiating different flagging pathways. Regarding the maturing interaction and the improvement of degenerative issues it appears to be that the main pathway entrained by insulin/IGF-1 is the standard phosphatidylinositol 3-kinase and serine–threonine protein kinases (Akt-1/Akt-2/protein kinase B [PKB]) flagging course. In C. elegans, this pathway decides reactions to life span and natural pressure. Transformations in C. elegans which inactivate the insulin/IGF-I pathway, including Daf-2, the receptor for insulin/IGF-I or the PI3K ortholog Age-1, increment life-range just as temperature and oxidative anxieties. These impacts require inversion of negative guideline of the pressure obstruction factor, Daf-16. Daf-16 encodes a record factor containing a "forkhead" DNA restricting space. Overexpression of Daf-16 in worms or an ortholog in flies essentially broadens their life expectancy. Daf-16 directs the declaration of a variety of qualities engaged with xenobiotic digestion and stress obstruction. Mammalian homologs of Daf-16 fall into the group of FoxO factors. There are four primary gatherings of mammalian FoxOs, FoxO1, FoxO3, FoxO4 and FoxO6. FoxO record factors have a place with the bigger Forkhead group of proteins, a group of transcriptional controllers portrayed by the preserved 'forkhead box' DNA-restricting area. These FoxO proteins control a wide cluster of qualities that all are connected by a typical component in that they serve to control energy metabolim in the organic entity because of ecological changes, for example limitation of accessible food. For instance FoxOs control qualities engaged with glucose digestion (glucose 6-phosphatase); cell passing (Fas-ligand), responsive oxygen species detoxification (catalse and manganese superoxide dismutase) and DNA fix (development capture and DNA harm inducible protein 45 and harm explicit DNA-restricting protein 1).

Insulin receptor incitement, during caloric admission, prompts enactment of the PI3K/Akt pathway and resultant phosphorylation of FoxOs in warm blooded animals. Phosphorylated FoxO factors are perceived by 14-3-3 proteins which work with their vehicle out of the core, decreasing their transcriptional action. Subsequently upon CR/IF there is an unpredictable transaction among enactment and inactivation of these FoxO factors. There are conceivably useful impacts of FoxO enactment and inactivation relying on the predominant cell conditions. Mammalian FoxO relatives complete capacities that decide cell endurance during seasons of pressure including guideline of apoptosis, cell-cycle designated spot control, and oxidative pressure opposition. Initiation of FoxO3 or FoxO4 prompts expansions in cell-cycle G1 capture and expansions in apoptosis probably as an approach to dispense with cells harmed by oxidative pressure. Hence changes in the ability to initiate the PI3K/Akt pathways can have emotional impacts upon cell survivability and this cycle might be basic in moving the beneficial outcomes of CR/IF to the living being. CR uncouples insulin/IGF-I motioning to FoxO factors by especially lessening plasma

IGF-I and insulin levels in subjects. These declines in coursing insulin/IGF-I levels result in diminished Akt phosphorylation in liver and diminished PI3K articulation in muscle. Moreover there is a compensatory expansion in the declaration of FoxO relatives by fasting or CR. Accordingly, when insulin flagging is diminished, for example during CR/IF there are expansions in atomic/cytoplasmic FoxO proportions however FoxO factor articulation also. By and large, numerous examinations have uncovered that down guideline of insulin/IGF-I flagging outcomes in expansions in the action of FoxO factors, that fundamentally direct cell endurance instruments, and that these changes are discovered reliably in numerous assorted models of life span among various species.

A significant number of the qualities directed by FoxOs are comparatively controlled by the tumor silencer p53, which has prompted the theory that these two qualities may work in show to forestall both injurious maturing and tumor development. Steady with this chance, p53 and FoxO are both phosphorylated and acetylated because of oxidative pressure boosts and UV radiations. Moreover, both p53 and FoxOs tie to SIRT1 deacetylase. FoxO and p53 appear to be practically connected as p53 can restrain FoxO work by actuating serum and glucocorticoid instigated kinase (SGK) - interceded phosphorylation of FoxO3 bringing about its movement from the core to the cytoplasm. FoxO3 has been found to forestall p53 from subduing SIRT1 quality articulation. FoxO-instigated suppression of p53 has all the earmarks of being interceded by the immediate cooperation somewhere in the range of FoxO3 and p53. That FoxO factors instigate SIRT1 articulation is steady with the perception that SIRT1 articulation is expanded in rat tissues when insulin and IGF-1 are brought down by CR. Thusly, SIRT1 itself can tie to and deacetylate p53 and FoxO record factors, controlling their movement. Subject holding a change, which brings about the actuation of p53, show a critical decrease of life expectancy and display indications of untimely maturing. Curiously, while initiation of p53 in these mouse models lessens life-range, p53 actuation actually permits an expanded protection from malignancy, exhibiting that p53 cause tumor concealment to the detriment of life span.

Perhaps the main ongoing fields of caloric limitation study is the exhibition that CR might have the option to forestall the age of various types of disease itself. For instance, in subject with hereditarily lessened p53 levels CR expanded the idleness of unconstrained tumor improvement (for the most part lymphomas) by around 75%. It is hence certain that there is an unobtrusive and confounded connection between these connected variables that are connected together by changes in dietary energy consumption.

Notwithstanding adverse guideline by insulin/IGF-1 flagging and p53, FoxO factors are managed by the CREB restricting protein (CBP) and a connected protein, p300. Curiously, cell overexpression of CBP or p300 improves the capacity of FoxO variables to actuate useful quality articulation. SIRT1 again appears to assume a focal part in versatile changes to energy guideline as it can turn around the negative guideline of FoxO relatives by CBP. Like PGC-1, SIRT1 levels are expanded during CR in subject liver and are contrarily directed by insulin and IGF-I. Moreover, the connected relative SIRT3, a mitochondrial protein, shows expanded articulation in white and earthy colored fat upon CR.

FoxOs appear to exist at a nexus between instruments that associate cell stress reactions to possible endurance components. For example the pressure related protein kinase cJun N-terminal kinase 1 (JNK-1), which fills in as an atomic sensor for different stressors effectively can handle FoxO transcriptional activity. In C. elegans, JNK-1 straightforwardly cooperates with and phosphorylates the FoxO homologue Daf-16, and because of warmth stress, JNK-1 advances the movement of Daf-16 into the core. Overexpression of JNK-1 in C. elegans prompts expansions in life-range and expanded endurance after heat pressure. In D. melanogaster also, gentle actuation of JNK prompts expanded pressure resilience and life span reliant upon a flawless FoxO.

Taking everything into account it appears to be that FoxO record factors are promising contender to fill in as sub-atomic connections between dietary adjustments and life span. In conditions like CR/IF where the flowing degrees of insulin/IGF-1 are constricted to improve euglycemia, FoxO atomic movement brings about the upregulation of a progression of target qualities that advance cell cycle capture, stress obstruction, and apoptosis. Outer distressing improvements additionally trigger the relocalization of FoxO factors into the core, subsequently permitting a versatile reaction to push upgrades. Steady with the idea that pressure opposition is profoundly combined with life-length expansion, actuation of FoxO record factors in worms and flies builds life span. FoxO proteins decipher natural upgrades, including the pressure initiated by caloric limitation into changes in quality articulation programs that may arrange organismal sound maturing and possible life span.

1.5 Intermittent Fasting and Caloric restriction in Humans

We are moving toward a complete comprehension of the different sub-atomic systems by which changes in caloric admission can be moved to an improved endurance of cells during the maturing cycle. Anyway the inquiry remains whether CR and IF will affect people. Until this point in time, there have been no all-around controlled logical examinations to decide the impacts of long haul CR on people. As of now there are considers progressing including 30% CR in non-human primates (rhesus monkeys) and information so distant from these investigations look encouraging, in that they have upheld the life-and wellbeing expanding properties of this dietary system.

In any case, the inordinate loss of muscle versus fat and the accompanying decrease in sex steroids can prompt feminine inconsistencies, amenorrhea, bone diminishing and the improvement of osteoporosis in females. Maybe a variety of the CR/IF conventions in which there is a milder caloric limitation joined with an adjustment of taking care of recurrence may have a more prominent probability of consistence among human subjects. Ideally this more delicate adjustment of dietary food admission will in any case hold the advantages of the trial systems utilized up until now. It is important that to date most examinations utilizing CR have contrasted the gainful impacts of CR with overweight (or even fat) age-coordinated with control creatures. It is muddled whether creatures with a sound bodyweight, that can participate in normal exercise and have some type of mental incitement (as they would do in the wild), would profit by a CR system. Ongoing investigations did with human subjects, subject to 25% CR, are anyway endeavoring to address this as they are utilizing control subjects with ordinary weight records.

The advancement of a substance CR mimetic might be a promising helpful road for the treatment of neurodegenerative illnesses and to defer the maturing cycle, as it would give comparative medical advantages to CR, (for example, expanding wellbeing and life expectancy), while going around the drawn out need to lessen food consumption. Notwithstanding, it stays not yet clear whether a CR mimetic would be a doable medication to deliver, particularly since the enthusiasm for the cycles whereby CR applies its defensive impacts are still fairly deficient and the fundamental components are ending up being perplexing. One should likewise not markdown the mental impacts of food admission in higher, more contemplative, creatures like people. We have a practically special enthusiastic association with an enormous assortment of staples. Consequently expulsion of this mental help, during a CR/IF-like system may mostly balance the physiological advantages of these ideal models.

The principle factor that may invalidate the far reaching execution of CR/IF as a compelling geronto-remedial is possibly the advanced Western way of life of close to steady work and industriously high feelings of anxiety. Henceforth, to fabricate the general public and innovative advances that we are utilized to, we have left behind the taking care of examples of our old progenitors for steady mental movement and restricted actual exercise. Because of expansions in our everyday movement we have an expanded energy (predominantly glucose) necessity while our physiology is generally still equipped to a dining experience and starvation example of energy consumption normal for our agrarian Homo sapiens precursors. This difficulty between our advanced society/conduct and our antiquated physiology will address a common issue for gerontology for quite a long time to come. Ideally, with our quickly propelling enthusiasm for our maturing interaction we won't have to trust that our physiological advancement will find our way of life.

Chapter 2. Intermittent Fasting and Reduced Meal Frequency

In spite of the fact that utilization of 3 suppers/d is the most widely recognized example of eating in industrialized nations, a logical reasoning for this feast recurrence regarding ideal wellbeing is deficient. An eating routine with less supper recurrence can improve the wellbeing and expand the life expectancy of research facility creatures, yet its impact on people has never been tried. A pilot study was directed to build up the impacts of a decreased dinner recurrence diet on wellbeing markers in solid, typical weight grown-ups. The examination was a randomized hybrid plan with two multi week treatment periods. During the treatment time frames, subjects devoured the entirety of the calories required for weight upkeep in either 3 suppers/d or 1 feast/d.

2.1 Introduction

Gorging is a significant reason for dreariness and mortality in people, and, likewise, caloric limitation has different medical advantages for the large. Caloric limitation may likewise improve the strength of people who are not viewed as overweight. While supplement thick, low-calorie eats less carbs have various medical advantages, the impact of dinner recurrence on wellbeing has not been set up. In any case, investigations of different research center creatures and explicitly of subjects have shown that dietary limitation (caloric limitation or intermittent fasting long haul intermittent fasting on account of subjects) can expand life expectancy and secure against or stifle infection measures liable for cardiovascular sickness (CVD), disease, diabetes, and neurodegenerative issues. The last investigations showed valuable impacts of intermittent fasting on circulatory strain, glucose digestion, and weakness of cardiovascular and synapses to injury. Notwithstanding an overall insight among people in general everywhere that it is critical to eat 3 dinners/d, no controlled investigations have straightforwardly looked at the impacts of various feast frequencies on human wellbeing. This information hole has been recognized by the 2005 Dietary Guidelines Advisory Committee Report as a future exploration heading.

Investigations of subjects and monkeys have prompted a few theories concerning the cell and atomic systems whereby dietary limitation expands life expectancy and ensures against infection. The oxidative pressure speculation recommends that maturing and age-related sicknesses result from combined oxidative harm to proteins, lipids, and nucleic acids; by diminishing the measure of oxyradicals delivered in mitochondria, dietary limitation impedes maturing and illness. A subsequent theory is that dietary limitation is helpful principally due to its impacts on energy digestion; i.e., it expands insulin affectability. A third speculation, which may have a specific connection to the useful impacts of diminished dinner recurrence/intermittent fasting, is that dietary limitation actuates a gentle cell stress reaction in which cells up-manage the statement of qualities that empower them to adapt to serious pressure. A few physiologic factors have been appeared to change in creatures kept up on caloric limitation or intermittent fasting regimens (or both), including diminished plasma insulin and glucose fixations, diminished circulatory strain and pulse, and improved invulnerable capacity. The current pilot study was directed to decide the attainability of controlled supper recurrence in ordinary weight, moderately aged people. A few physiologic results and biomarkers of wellbeing were likewise examined.

2.2 Methods and Subjects

Sound people matured 40–50 y were enlisted by paper ad from the more prominent Washington, DC, metropolitan region. Incorporation in the investigation depended on a weight record (BMI; in kg) somewhere in the range of 18 and 25 and a typical eating example of 3 dinners/d. Subjects were rejected on the off chance that they detailed tobacco use, late pregnancy or lactation, history of CVD or drug use for CVD, hypertension, diabetes, mental condition, malignancy, or work in high-hazard occupations (this last avoidance basis was because of the potential for wooziness or shortcoming during the dinner skipping stage). Study passage was endorsed by a doctor based on clinical history, blood and pee test screening results, and an actual assessment.

Study Design

This examination was a randomized hybrid plan with two multi week treatment periods. During the treatment time frames, subjects burned-through the entirety of their calories for weight support circulated in either 3 dinners/d (control diet) or 1 supper/d (test diet). A multi week waste of time period was incorporated between medicines. The control diet comprised of 3 suppers/d (breakfast, lunch, and supper) and the test "dinner skipping" (or 1 feast/d) diet comprised of a similar every day allocation of food eaten inside a 4 hours' time frame in the early evening. The subjects were taken care of at an energy consumption that would keep up body weight so feast recurrence would be the lone significant change in their eating routine over the span of the investigation. The examination was a communitarian exertion between the US Department of Agriculture, Beltsville Human Nutrition Research Center (BHNRC; Beltsville, MD), and the National Institute on Aging.

Study Diets

Every day, subjects burned-through supper at the BHNRC Human Study Facility under the oversight of an enlisted dietitian. Toward the finish of supper, subject dinner plate were examined to guarantee total utilization of the food. All morning meals and snacks were pressed for complete. Just food sources given by the Human Study Facility were permitted to be devoured during the examination. A 7 days menu pattern of ordinary

American food varieties was detailed by utilizing nutritionist.

During the initial fourteen days of the investigation, subjects haphazardly appointed to the 1 supper/d eating routine were taken care of 2 dinners/d (lunch and supper); for the following a month and a half, all food was burned-through somewhere in the range of 1700 and 2100, which made a base quick of 20 h/d. While keeping up the equivalent macronutrient dissemination among test and control diets, breakfast and lunch food things were fill in for customary evening feast things. Energy-thick food varieties were picked to help with decreasing the volume of food to be burned-through.

Subjects were permitted limitless measures of sans calorie food varieties like water, espresso (without sugar or milk), diet sodas, salt, and pepper. A multi day crisis supply of food that met the examination convention was given to each expose to use during any severe climate. Subjects were needed to burn-through the entirety of the food sources and just the food varieties given by the Human Study Facility at determined occasions during the controlled taking care of periods.

Body weight was estimated each day prior to the evening supper, when subjects showed up at the office. So that subjects could keep up consistent body weight during the investigation, energy admission was changed in 200-kcal increases. Energy prerequisites for weight upkeep were determined by utilizing the Harris-Benedict recipe, which gauges basal energy use, and duplicated by a movement factor of 1.3–1.5. This recipe has demonstrated effective in assessing weight-upkeep energy necessities at our office. Subjects finished an everyday poll in regards to their overall wellbeing; any utilization of remedy or over-the-counter prescriptions; factors identified with dietary consistence; and exercise played out; the survey likewise offered subjects the chance to write in inquiries of their own about the eating regimen. Subjects were urged to keep up their ordinary exercise routine all through the examination.

Physiologic Evaluations

Physiologic factors estimated were pulse, pulse, internal heat level, and body piece. These estimations were gathered at standard, a month, and toward the finish of every one of the 2 treatment time frames. Momentarily, subjects were situated in a tranquil space for 5 min, and circulatory strain and pulse were estimated multiple times with a Dinamap Compact Monitor. Internal heat level was estimated on either a Dinamap or a compact oral computerized thermometer. Body organization was estimated by utilizing bioelectrical impedance investigation (BIA). Subjects abstained and avoided substantial exercise before these estimations. Abstract satiety and appetite were evaluated day by day before utilization of the evening dinner, in both the trial and control slims down, by utilizing 4 visual simple scales (VASs) that depicted yearning, want to eat, the measure of food that could be eaten, and stomach completion. The VASs were every one of the 100-mm long, and they were moored at one or the flip side with terms demonstrating inverse descriptors.

Analysis of Biological Sample

Blood was gathered at benchmark, a month, and the finish of every one of the 2 treatment time frames after at least 12 h of fasting. The entirety of the standard examples were gathered in the first part of the day. The a month and end-of-treatment tests were gathered toward the beginning of the day from subjects following the control diet and in the evening (before supper) from subjects following the 1 feast/d eating regimen. Also, as a proportion of consistence, blood tests were gathered at unannounced occasions on 3 events from the subjects when they were burning-through 1 supper/d and were broke down for fasting blood glucose and triacylglycerol focuses. The gathered blood tests were utilized to plan 0.8–2.0-mL aliquots of plasma, serum, and red platelets that were put away at short 80 °C in cryovials. Test examinations incorporated a lipid profile, an extensive metabolic board, and total blood tally (CBC), and cortisol fixation. Investigations were performed at the Core Laboratory of the public foundations of wellbeing) and at clinical lab by utilizing standard strategies and quality-control measures from the clinical research facility improvement changes. Plasma absolute cholesterol, HDL cholesterol, and triacylglycerol were estimated enzymatically with business units on 250 analyzer. LDL-cholesterol focuses were determined by utilizing the condition. Serum cortisol focuses were investigated on an immunoassay analyzer (with CVs of 5.3% and 7.2%, individually).

Assessment of Physical Activity

Actual work observing (PAM) was surveyed with the utilization of the Actigraph accelerometer throughout 7 days to acquire the normal day by day and week by week action checks. Estimations were acquired during week 2 (benchmark) and week 7 (finish of treatment) of every treatment period. Subjects were told to wear the movement screen as long as conceivable consistently. The movement screen, worn as a cozily fitting belt around the midriff with the producer's "score" confronting vertically, was set to peruse the information in 1-min portions. Subjects were approached to wear the screen on the correct hip, except if they revealed being not able to do as such. Notwithstanding the action screen position, each subject wore the screen on a similar side and at a similar area all through the examination. As well as wearing the screens, subjects kept a little day by day log to detail the occasions when the screen was worn, the exercises that were done when the screen was not worn (i.e., dozing or showering), and any activity performed (if the screen was worn). In every one of the treatment time frames, subjects were approached to wear the screen for 9 days, fully intent on getting 7 entire long periods of information. In the event that a subject detailed not wearing the action screen for a given day, the person in question was approached to wear the screen an additional day.

Active work information got from the Actigraph accelerometer were handled by utilizing a strategy created in our office. Momentarily, most subjects commonly eliminate the screens occasionally during the day or around evening time for rest (or both). Investigations from our lab show that these missing information focuses can detrimentally affect the forecast of active work, so we built up a methodology that treats each checking day as a 24-hours day regardless of how long the screen was worn on quickly. Screen records are filtered by a program that assesses the time spent dozing and credits a consistent incentive for those occasions. Other missing strings of information 20 min long are "filled in" by attribution, based on the screen evacuation times announced in the log. These information preparing strategies significantly diminish the inconstancy intrinsic with movement screen information.

Analysis of Stats

An examination of change (ANOVA) fitting for a 2-period hybrid investigation with rehashed measures inside period was utilized to assess supper recurrence impacts on result factors utilizing the blended method in programming. The factual model included grouping, supper recurrence, period, time inside period, and time duplicate by feast recurrence collaboration as fixed impacts. Period and time were displayed as rehashed measures. The factor subject settled in grouping was remembered for the model as an intermittent impact. The primary perception inside a period was incorporated as a covariate. At the point when the time multiply by dinner recurrence connection was critical (P is equivalent to 0.05), inside time supper recurrence impacts were assessed by utilizing rehashed measures ANOVA. In the event that this collaboration was not huge, the principle impact of dinner recurrence was assessed. Information are introduced as means SEMs.

Characteristics of Subjects

69 people went to the examination data meeting. 35 gave composed educated assent, and 32 finished the screening interaction. 21 subjects (14 ladies, 7 men) at last were haphazardly appointed to the medicines. Fifteen subjects (10 ladies, 5 men) finished the taking care of period of the investigation. Complete information were examined and are introduced for 15 subjects. In the 3 feast/d eating routine arm, 1 subject pulled out in light of food disdains. During the 1 feast/d eating regimen, 5 subjects pulled out in light of booking clashes and medical issues irrelevant to the examination. Just 1 of the 5 subjects pulled out explicitly due to a reluctance to devour the 1 supper/d eating regimen. The mean BMI showed that subjects were inside the ordinary reach. The actual qualities of the 15 subjects at gauge are introduced.

Diet Plans

The sythesis of the 2 weight control plans is appeared. Subject adherence to the controlled eating regimens was decided to be great based on noticed utilization of the suppers in the office and audit of the reactions on the day by day surveys. The intermittent fasting triacylglycerol and glucose focuses demonstrated that consistence with the 1 feast/d eating regimen was worthy. The mean triacylglycerol and glucose fixations were 64.4 and 79.7 mg/dL, individually. Thirty of 1650 evening dinners (1.8%) gave during the whole examination were stuffed for utilization away from the office. The normal day by day energy admission across medicines was 2364 kcal in the 1 dinner/d eating regimen and 2429 kcal in the 3 suppers/d eating routine. No huge contrasts were found in the rates of macronutrients, unsaturated fats, cholesterol, and fiber between the 2 controlled eating regimens.

Blood Pressure

Systolic and diastolic blood pressures were essentially brought down by 6% during the period when subjects were devouring 3 dinners/d than when they were burning-through 1 supper/day. No critical impact of time (estimations taken at week 4 and week 8) or of treatment arrangement on circulatory strain was seen. No critical contrasts in pulse and internal heat level were seen between the 2 eating routine regimens.

Scales of Visual Analogue

There was a huge treatment impact between the 2 weight control plans on evaluations of appetite, want to eat, completion, and forthcoming utilization (i.e., the measure of food subjects figured they could eat). The 1 dinner/d eating routine was altogether higher for hunger (P is equivalent to 0.003), want to eat (P is equivalent to 0.004), and planned utilization (P is equivalent to 0.006) than was the 3 suppers/d eating regimen. Sensations of completion were essentially (P is equivalent to 0.001) lower in the 1 feast/day than in the 3 dinners/day diet. Notwithstanding the huge treatment impact by diet, a huge time impact (day of study) was noticed for hunger, want to eat, totality, and imminent utilization. Over the long run, hunger, want to eat, and imminent utilization were fundamentally higher in the 1 dinner/day than in the 3 suppers/day diet. Completion was fundamentally lower over the long run in the 1 supper/day diet than in the 3 dinners/day diet.

Body Composition and Weight

Subjects' weight and muscle versus fat mass were brought down (1.4 and 2.1 kg, separately) after utilization of the 1 supper/day diet yet not after utilization of the 3 dinners/day diet. No critical contrasts in sans fat mass and complete body water were seen between the eating routine gatherings. Indeed, even with an 11-week waste of time period between the 2 eating routine conventions, no critical contrasts from benchmark were found in body weight, fat mass, sans fat mass, or complete body water in one or the other time of the investigation. No proof was found of a critical contrast in active work after utilization of the 1 supper/day or the 3 dinners/day diet.

Biological Samples

Utilization of 1 dinner/day brought down blood urea nitrogen by 13.4%. The serum liver proteins antacid phosphatase, serum glutamic pyruvic transaminase, and serum glutamic oxaloacetic transaminase were higher 4.6%, 17.5%, and 16.0% higher, individually, when subjects devoured 1 feast/day than when they burned-through 3 dinners/d. Serum egg whites was 4.5% higher and cortisol fixations were 48.9% lower after utilization of 1 dinner/day than after utilization of 3 suppers/day. Aggregate, LDL, and HDL cholesterol were 11.7%, 16.8%, and 8.4% higher, separately, in subjects devouring 1 supper/day than in those burning-through 3 dinners/day. The hematologic factors that contrasted altogether between the eating regimens bunches were those of hemoglobin, hematocrit and red platelets. Serum convergences of creatinine, glucose, complete protein, uric corrosive, and any remaining metabolic factors were not essentially influenced by the weight control plans.

2.4 Discussion

This investigation is among the main controlled randomized clinical preliminaries to assess the impacts of controlled feast recurrence on ordinary weight, moderately aged grown-ups. We tracked down that the utilization of a dinner skipping diet (i.e., 1 supper/day), instead of the customary 3 dinners/day diet, is attainable for a brief length.

Our examination withdrawal rate was 28.6%. Commonplace paces of withdrawal from human taking care of studies at our office are 4–7% (18–20). We can estimate that subject withdrawals expanded on the grounds that the subjects were approached to devour all nourishment for the day in 1 dinner; nonetheless, just 1 subject explicitly expressed this justification pulling out. Most subjects had the option to burn-through all calories in the 1 feast/day diet. Study withdrawals were accounted for to be because of subject booking clashes and medical conditions that were irrelevant to the investigation.

A couple of exploratory investigations have tried the impact of feast recurrence on satiety measures. The aftereffects of the VASs recommend that subjects didn't get acclimated to the 1 dinner/day diet. Over the long run, hunger, want to eat, and forthcoming utilization expanded, while sensations of completion diminished. Essentially, subjects who followed another day-fasting diet for multi week had a critical expansion in craving and want to eat on their fasting days than at gauge, however they didn't get acclimated to the other day-fasting diet, and they were similarly as eager on their first day of fasting as on the most recent day. Albeit abstract craving and satiety evaluations were not made after the evening supper, in remarks during utilization of the 1 feast/day diet, most subjects detailed limit totality after the dinner and experienced issues completing their food in the assigned time. Further exploration is needed to acquire a superior comprehension of emotional satiety on dinner recurrence.

In spite of the fact that inside typical qualities, both systolic and diastolic blood pressures were higher than pattern during utilization of the 1 feast/day diet. Trial information for typical weight people on the impacts of utilization of 1 feast/day instead of 3 dinners/day on pulse have not recently been accounted for. Overweight people showed that utilization of 1 supper/day, with caloric limitation, improved circulatory strain and pulse after work out. In creature models, intermittent fasting without caloric limitation has been appeared to diminish pulse and pulse. The noticed expansion in pulse in our subject populace burning-through 1 feast/day might be because of a circadian cadence in circulatory strain. Diurnal changes may have happened, in light of the fact that pulse estimations were acquired in the late evening in the 1 dinner/d eating routine versus early morning in the 3 suppers/day.

It is fascinating that body weight and muscle versus fat diminished in the 1 supper/day diet, which might be mostly clarified by a slight shortfall of 65 kcal in day by day energy admission. This adjustment of body organization may likewise be impacted by the impact that eating examples could have on metabolic action. Subjects that followed a snacking diet and afterward an eating routine that comprising of 1 enormous dinner built up an expansion net transition of free unsaturated fats from fat stores and an increment in gluconeogenesis. Comparable changes in digestion may have happened in our subjects, which may have added to weight and fat mass misfortune. Gluconeogenesis ordinarily starts 4–6 hours after the last feast and turns out to be completely dynamic as stores of liver glycogen are exhausted. Free unsaturated fats and amino acids that are substrates for gluconeogenesis are utilized for the energy supply.

Adjusted coursing lipid focuses are perceived as hazard factors for CVD. In the current investigation, we found both (expansions altogether and LDL cholesterol) and (an increment in HDL cholesterol and a reduction in triacylglycerols) changes after utilization of the 1 dinner/day diet. These progressions gave off an impression of being autonomous of the controlled eating regimens, since dietary cholesterol and the proportion of unsaturated fats were held steady. Studies that have endeavored to decide the impacts of supper recurrence on biomarkers of wellbeing, like lipid focuses, are conflicting. In one exploratory investigation, sound men were taken care of either 3 dinners/day or 17 little bites/d for multi week; subjects burning-through the 17-nibble diet had decreases altogether and LDL-cholesterol fixations, while the focuses didn't change in the subjects burning-through 3 suppers/day. Two examinations likewise showed that excluding breakfast effect wellbeing results identified with CVD, and another investigation showed that this exclusion may diminish hazard factors for CVD.

Utilization of 1 feast/d expanded egg whites and liver catalysts and diminished blood urea nitrogen in our examination subjects, albeit these qualities stayed inside typical reference ranges. Subjects burning-through the 1 feast/d eating regimen additionally had diminished cortisol focuses. Albeit all blood assortment happened following 12 hours of fasting, the circumstance of blood assortment contrasted between the 2 eating regimen gatherings. Blood was gathered in the early morning, before breakfast (i.e., following a 12 hours quick), from subjects burning-through 3 suppers/day and in the late evening, before the evening feast (i.e., following a 18-hours quick), from those burning-through I dinner/day. Subjects burning-through 1 dinner/day had diminished cortisol fixations, which were in all probability because of diurnal varieties in this chemical. Cortisol is ordinarily raised in the first part of the day and diminishes later in the early evening.

During Ramadan, the heavenly month during which Muslims quick from day break to nightfall, diurnal varieties of nourishment biomarkers have been seen in rehearsing Muslims. Past research has shown that, dissimilar to in non-fasting periods, cortisol focuses are biphasic during Ramadan fasting. These specialists announced an increment in serum cortisol beginning at 1200 hours that arrives at a level somewhere in the range of 1600 and 2000. During Ramadan fasting, diurnal variety in cortisol varies altogether from the ordinary diurnal variety. We found that subjects' hemoglobin, hematocrit, and red platelets were lower after utilization of the 1 supper/day diet, while the mean cell volume was viewed as of ordinary focus. The last outcomes could be the consequence of an expansion in blood volume or an adjustment of the creation of red platelets. Past research on Ramadan fasting has shown a concealment in red platelet creation alongside an expanding pattern for pallor. The last outcomes were likely because of a reduction in the admissions of calories and of iron-containing food varieties during the fasting month of Ramadan. No major, clinically pertinent, diet-related changes were found in the exhaustive metabolic board or CBC, which demonstrated that the 1 dinner/day diet was very much endured in that gathering of solid people.

A few impediments of the plan of the current examination warrant thought. Albeit this was a pilot study, the little example size was especially restricting. Blood, circulatory strain, internal heat level, and body-piece estimations were taken in the early morning from subjects devouring 3 dinners/day and in the late evening from those burning-through I feast/day; results may have varied if the last estimations additionally were gotten in the early morning. BIA may likewise not be the best technique for evaluating body organization due to its inclination to overestimate fat mass in fit subjects. The subject populace of the flow concentrate additionally was genuinely homogenous; future exploration ought to incorporate overweight and stout populaces to permit assurance of the impacts of feast recurrence in those gatherings.

Past examinations archived enhancements in the wellbeing and life span of subjects and subject kept up on an intermittent fasting routine wherein they were denied of nourishment for a 24-hours' time frame each and every day; in these investigations, the test diet brought about by and large decreases in calorie admission of up to 30%. Nonetheless, in certain investigations, the measure of caloric limitation was little (5–10%) and the physiologic changes were generally huge, which recommends that the all-inclusive fasting period itself added to the advantages of the eating regimen. The current discoveries propose that, without a decrease in calorie consumption, a diminished dinner recurrence diet doesn't bear the cost of significant medical advantages in people. Enhancements in glucose guideline and cardiovascular wellbeing in subjects happen during a while of intermittent fasting; the time during which the subjects were kept up on the 1 supper/day diet in the current investigation may in this manner not be adequate to accomplish stable changes in physiology. A drawn out diminished dinner recurrence diet that likewise remembers a 20–30% decrease for calorie admission would all the more intently look like the intermittent fasting routine that is broadly utilized in rat contemplates.

Taking everything into account, changed supper recurrence is possible in sound, typical weight, moderately aged people. Utilization of 1 supper/day brought about weight reduction and a lessening in fat mass with little alteration in calorie utilization. It stays indistinct whether adjusted feast recurrence would prompt changes in weight and body synthesis in large subjects.

Chapter 3. Intermittent Fasting and Neuronal Resistance to Injury from Calorie Intake

Dietary limitation has been appeared to have a few medical advantages including expanded insulin affectability, stress obstruction, decreased dismalness, and expanded life expectancy. The component stays obscure, however the requirement for a drawn out decrease in caloric admission to accomplish these advantages has been accepted. We report that when subject are kept up on an intermittent fasting (substitute day fasting) dietary-limitation routine their general food admission isn't diminished and their body weight is kept up. All things considered, intermittent fasting brought about useful impacts that met or surpassed those of caloric limitation including diminished serum glucose and insulin levels and expanded opposition of neurons in the cerebrum to excitotoxic stress. Intermittent fasting accordingly effects glucose guideline and neuronal protection from injury in these subject that are autonomous of caloric admission.

3.1 Introduction

Maturing alludes to the organic changes that happen during a lifetime that outcome in decreased protection from stress, expanded weakness to sickness, and an expanded likelihood of death. The rate at which maturing happens is species-explicit, proposing a solid hereditary impact. The solitary natural variable that has been appeared to especially influence the pace of maturing in a wide scope of animal categories is caloric admission: Restricting food admission to a level underneath that which would be burned-through intentionally brings about an abatement in the pace of maturing and an expansion in normal and greatest life expectancy. Dietary limitation (DR) decreases malignancy arrangement and kidney infection and builds the opposition of neurons to brokenness and degeneration in exploratory models of Alzheimer's and Parkinson's sicknesses just as stroke. Two diverse DR standards have demonstrated powerful in expanding life expectancy and infection opposition in subjects and subject. In one worldview creatures are given a day by day food allocation that is regularly 30–40% not exactly the not obligatory (AL) utilization of a control populace; this restricted day by day taking care of (LDF) worldview includes a controlled caloric limitation and a comparing decrease in body weight. In the second worldview creatures are exposed to intermittent (substitute day) fasting (IF), which in subjects brings about diminished food admission after some time and diminished body weight.

Confining caloric admission makes the limited populace weigh relatively not exactly the AL-took care of gathering. Undoubtedly, weight decrease commonly somewhat surpasses the level of food limitation, so food consumption per gram of body weight is accounted for reliably to be marginally higher in LDF creatures than in their AL-took care of partners. Subjects and subject typically shed pounds when kept up on an IF routine, albeit a few strains, for example, subject may lose practically no weight. Both the IF and LDF ideal models are accounted for to bring about emotional expansions in life length in contrast with AL-took care of creatures, however little else is known concerning the likenesses and contrasts in their belongings.

It appears to be sensible to expect that both LDF and IF standards of DR expand life range through a typical instrument. To acquire knowledge into the idea of the basic component, we analyzed the impacts of LDF and IF eats less on a few boundaries that have been hypothesized to assume a part in the defensive impacts of DR including body weight, food admission, and fasting levels of serum insulin, glucose, and insulin-like development factor 1 (IGF-1). Furthermore, ongoing investigations have shown that subjects and subject kept up on an IF routine display expanded obstruction of neurons in their minds to affronts applicable to the pathogenesis of a few distinctive human neurological problems including epileptic seizures and stroke. We thusly played out an analysis to decide if LDF and IF consumes less calories apply comparable advantageous consequences for neurons in the mind.

3.2 Methods

Measurement of Food Intake

Six-week-old subject were gotten from Charles River Breeding Laboratories, housed in the National Institute on Aging Gerontology Research Center creature state, and took care of a standard eating routine. Food was given AL until 9 weeks old enough. Around then, subject were appointed to one of three gatherings: AL, taken care of not indispensable; IF, gave admittance to food each and every other day; and LDF, furnished with a restricted day by day food distribution of 60% of that eaten by the AL-took care of creatures. To control for caloric admission versus occasional food hardship, a fourth gathering was added: These pair-took care of (PF) subject were given day by day a food assignment equivalent to the normal day by day admission of subject in the IF bunch. Water was accessible AL for all gatherings. The creatures were kept in a 12-hours light/12-hours dull cycle (lights on at 6 a.m. what's more, off at 6 p.m.); food was given or taken out at 10 a.m. Body weight was resolved every week around the same time and time. Food admission was estimated day by day. To monitor spillage, white sheet material was utilized to permit simple partition of unconsumed food and powder from waste and bedding; spilled food was permitted to dry completely to stay away from estimation of wet weight added by pee. Measurable correlations were made by utilizing ANOVA. All systems were supported by the public establishment on maturing gerontology research focus creature care and use board.

Collection and Analysis of Blood

At 29 weeks old enough, all subject were abstained for 14 hours before blood withdrawal. Blood was taken out by means of intraorbital seep under isoflurane sedation, and serum was separated. In primer investigations we tracked down that the glucose fixations in blood tests from abstained subject gathered following the subject surrender to the isoflurane inward breath sedation (inside 1 min of openness to the sedative) are basically indistinguishable from the glucose focuses in blood tests from abstained subject killed by execution inside 10 seconds of expulsion from their confine. The groupings of glucose and insulin were controlled by utilizing the glucose oxidase technique and RIA, individually. IGF-1 focuses were dictated by utilizing a chemical immunosorbent test pack, and beta-hydroxybutyrate fixations were controlled by utilizing examine that actions the oxidation of beta-hydroxybutyrate to acetoacetate by utilizing a unit bought from Sigma. Measurable correlations were made by utilizing single-factor ANOVA; if critical, pairwise examinations were made by utilizing a two-followed t test expecting inconsistent change.

Administration and Quantification

Subject were treated at 30–38 weeks old enough. Kainate was infused into the dorsal part of the correct hippocampus by utilizing the techniques portrayed. Momentarily, subject were anesthetized with Avertin and put in a stereotaxic head holder, and the skull was uncovered along the midline. A light portion of kainate was infused singularly into the dorsal hippocampus (stereotaxic arranges were 2.0 mm back to bregma, 2.4 mm sidelong to bregma, and 1.8 mm underneath the outside of the skull). The contralateral hippocampus of each mouse got an infusion of 0.5 miniature liter of PBS. 24 hours after kainate organization, subject were anesthetized with isoflurane and perfused transcardially with saline followed by cool phosphate-cushioned 4% paraformaldehyde. Coronal cerebrum segments were cut on a freezing microtome and stained with violet. Positive intact neurons were included in three duplicate 40 fields in areas CA3 and CA1. Includes were made in five coronal cerebrum areas for every mouse (segments were picked by fair testing), and the mean number of cells per segment was resolved with the end goal that the worth got for every creature addresses a normal all out number of neurons tallied per segment (i.e., amount of six duplicate 40 fields for each hippocampal locale). Examinations of quantities of intact neurons in hippocampal districts among treatment bunches were made by utilizing ANOVA followed by post hoc and tests for pairwise correlations.

3.3 Results

Before the finish of this investigation, male subject exposed to IF were burning-through basically similar measure of food in a 48-hours' time frame as did those took care of AL. When they approached food, the IF subject ate generally twice as much as did subject took care of AL. Subject on the LDF routine devoured 40% less food as given: this was reflected in their body loads, which were 49% lower than those of the AL-took care of gathering. Conversely, toward the finish of the examination the body loads of subject

71

kept up on the IF diet or PF consistently were just somewhat underneath those of the AL-took care of gathering. An unmistakable physiological change that happens in warm blooded creatures kept up on diminished calorie consumes less calories is expanded insulin affectability, which frequently is reflected in diminished fasting plasma levels of glucose and insulin. Fasting serum convergences of glucose and insulin in subject took care of AL in the current examination found the middle value of 150 mg/dl and 3,400 pg/ml, separately. The convergences of glucose and insulin were diminished essentially, to comparable sums, in subject kept up on either LDF or IF regimens with glucose and insulin focuses dropping to 100 mg/dl and 700–1,100 pg/ml, separately. That comparable changes are seen in IF and LDF bunches in the current examination recommends that in spite of a general calorie admission like subject took care of AL, IF effect coursing glucose and insulin levels.

Male subject make up for times of fasting by expanding their food admission and putting on weight at rates like subject took care of AL. Shown are the normal every day food admissions (determined from 14-day consumption) (a) and body loads (b) in subject kept up on one of four taking care of regimens: AL, IF, PF, and LDF (40% decrease in calories comparative with AL-took care of). On the off chance that body loads are post taking care of qualities. Qualities are the mean of estimations made in eight subject for every eating routine gathering. Toward the finish of the investigation, body loads and food admissions of the LDF bunch were fundamentally lower than the body loads and food admissions of the AL-took care of and IF gatherings (P under 0.001 for each situation). Body loads and food admissions of the AL-took care of and IF bunches were not altogether extraordinary.

Levels of circling IGF-1 were diminished in subject on the LDF diet however expanded in subject on the IF diet. These discoveries are of impressive interest considering proof that the insulin flagging pathway is connected to life span in an assortment of animal varieties, and that IGF-1 levels are decreased in subjects on calorie-limited eating regimens. Since subject on the IF routine were not calorie-limited, the distinction in IGF-1 levels between the IF and LDF bunches recommends a distinction in the manners by which IF and caloric limitation impact the development chemical (GH)– IGF-1 hub and insulin flagging pathways. Since insulin levels were diminished in IF subject to levels even lower than in LDF subject, these two DR regimens uncover a separation in the instruments managing IGF-1 and insulin levels. Transgenic subjects with diminished degrees of GH display a transgene portion subordinate decrease in degrees of IGF-1; subjects with a moderate decrease in IGF-1 levels live more, though those with a more prominent abatement in IGF-1 levels have a diminished life expectancy. The last outcomes recommend that there is an ideal level of the GH–IGF-1 hub to augment endurance in vertebrates. Concerning the neuroprotective impacts of IF (see information underneath and refs. 6–9), contemplates have announced that IGF-1 flagging is neuroprotective in trial models of neurodegenerative issues. It will be of extensive interest in this manner to decide the systems by which LDF and IF differentially influence IGF-1 levels and insulin flagging and how these progressions impact energy digestion, life span, and infection obstruction.

Fasting is known to bring about an expanded creation of ketone bodies, which can be utilized as a fuel source and are known to give some defensive impacts including neuroprotection and protection from epileptic seizures. We hence estimated serum levels of beta-hydroxybutyrate after an overnight quick in subject that had been kept up on AL, LDF, and IF counts calories. Subject on the IF diet showed a 2-overlay expansion in the fasting serum centralization of beta-hydroxybutyrate contrasted and subject took care of AL. interestingly, the beta-hydroxybutyrate convergence of subject on the LDF diet were diminished contrasted and subject took care of AL.

When the excitotoxin kainic corrosive (KA) is infused into the dorsal hippocampus of subject it instigates seizures and harm to pyramidal neurons in locales CA3 and CA1. KA was infused into the dorsal hippocampus of subject that had been kept up for 24 weeks on AL, LDF, and IF abstains from food. All subject displayed captures of comparable greatness and span (information not appeared). Subject were killed 24 hours after KA organization, tissue areas from their cerebrums were stained with violet, and the quantities of neurons in locales CA3 and CA1 of every hippocampus were checked. KA caused a stamped deficiency of CA3 and CA1 neurons in subject took care of AL. True to form, numerous neurons in districts CA3 and CA1 of the hippocampus infused with KA declined. There was a huge expansion in the endurance of CA3 and CA1 neurons in the IF subject contrasted and subject took care of AL. LDF additionally assured the CA1 neurons, yet to a lesser sum than did IF, yet didn't ensure CA3 neurons against KA-initiated harm. Curiously, the subject PF to the IF bunch additionally showed an expanded obstruction of CA1 neurons to KA-actuated harm comparative with either AL-took care of or LDF subject. The significant contrast between the AL-took care of and PF bunches is that the last were marginally confined from the get-go in the examination (10%). This may infer that there is an ideal degree of limitation for neuroprotective impacts, a theory that would require further investigation to check. The 10% limitation in food admission of subject on the IF routine may represent the contrasts between AL-took care of and PF subject and furthermore might be a factor in the impacts of IF on some physiological boundaries in this examination.

In the event that is better than caloric limitation in securing hippocampal neurons against excitotoxic injury. Subject that had been kept up for 20 weeks on the showed abstains from food were exposed to an intrahippocampal infusion of the excitotoxin KA; PBS was infused into the contralateral hippocampus of each mouse. Subject were killed 24 hours after the fact, coronal cerebrum segments were stained with violet, and the quantities of whole neurons in locales CA3 and CA1 of the hippocampus were evaluated. Qualities are the mean and SD of judgments made in eight subject for every gathering. (a) Illustrations of violet-stained neurons in KA- and PBS-infused hippocampi of subject from each diet group. (b) Quantification of harm in hippocampi infused with PBS or KA.

A past report looked at the impacts of LDF and IF on life length in male C57BL/6 subject, with the two DR regimens bringing about comparative life expectancy expansion notwithstanding an unmistakable contrast in body weight between the two gatherings. Notwithstanding, food admission was not decided, and it was expected that the distinction in body weight was because of some factor other than caloric admission. The current investigation sets up that it is the capacity of this strain of subject to glut on days when food is given that permits them to keep up almost AL body weight when taken care of each and every other day, and they accordingly stay away from a drawn out calorie deficiency. That IF taking care of was more successful than either LDF or PF in shielding neurons from KA-instigated harm exhibits that the IF-taking care of timetable itself is neuroprotective autonomous of generally caloric admission. In an investigation of subjects found that when calories are expressly limited to 60% of the AL consumption, modifying dinner recurrence inside a 24-hours' time frame neither revokes nor improves the impact of the net caloric limitation on life length. Despite the fact that giving proof that supper recurrence doesn't adjust the capacity of caloric limitation to expand life range that review didn't permit an end with respect to whether IF can build life length free of by and large calorie admission. The current examination recommends that without express limitation, fasting may assume a part in probably a portion of the impacts of DR.

Since we didn't decide life length in this examination, we can't close with sureness that the IF routine utilized would broaden life range. Notwithstanding, a past report set up a life expectancy broadening impact of the indistinguishable IF routine in the indistinguishable strain of subject. Besides, a new investigation of subject with fat tissue-particular disturbance of the insulin receptor quality showed that the life expectancy of subject can be expanded without a decrease in calorie consumption. Arising information from this and different research facilities subsequently support future examinations to decide if a decrease in caloric admission is the solitary dietary strategy to build life span or whether IF without caloric limitation may have helpful impacts too. In this manner, albeit caloric limitation is one significant component fundamental the impacts of various DR regimens on life length and infection vulnerability, probably some valuable impacts of DR regimens may result from a system other than a general decrease in calorie consumption. One such conceivable component is incitement of cell stress-obstruction pathways, which are prompted firmly by the IF routine utilized in this investigation.

A predictable hormonal reaction to a diminishing in food consumption in subjects, nonhuman primates, and people is a decrease in insulin levels and an expansion in insulin affectability. We found that subject exposed to IF showed diminishes in serum levels of glucose and insulin to levels at or underneath those in subject took care of every day except with a 40% decrease in caloric admission. The capacity of IF to modify fasting levels of insulin and glucose was autonomous of by and large caloric admission. It has been recommended that some helpful impacts of DR result from diminished blood glucose levels (incorporated over the long haul). Glucose levels in the blood, incorporated over the long haul, have been proposed to prompt undeniable degrees of nonenzymatic glycation, a type of protein harm. Higher fuel accessibility may likewise prompt an expanded recurrence of mitochondrial state-four breath, with resulting expansions in receptive oxygen species creation from the mitochondrial respiratory chain. DR has been appeared to impact oxyradical creation and harm and nonenzymatic glycation. The current discoveries are predictable with a part for glucose in the advantageous impacts of IF, on the grounds that the creatures spend an enormous extent of their life expectancy in an abstained state. Notwithstanding, it very well may be anticipated that on taking care of days, when IF subject gorge on food, their degrees of oxyradical creation and glycation are a lot higher than in subject on the LDF routine. Evidently, restricting episodes of high caloric admission to a restricted time window with long mediating times of fasting brings about versatile reactions that don't happen when suppers are more successive. Past examinations have shown that there are huge changes in respiratory remainder as limited creatures move from ingested to put away fuel. It is possible that rotating times of anabolism and catabolism assume a robotic part in setting off expansions in cell stress opposition and the maintenance of harmed biomolecules or cells. Late discoveries recommend that a considerable lot of the valuable impacts of IF may result from a cell stress reaction actuated by the abstained state. For instance, it was shown that degrees of stress protein chaperones and neurotrophic factors are expanded in subjects and subject kept up on an IF-taking care of routine. The prevalent neuroprotective adequacy of IF contrasted and LDF taking care of archived in this investigation is predictable with improvement of cell stress obstruction that outcomes from the pressure related with fasting as opposed to a general decrease in caloric admission.

Strangely, despite the fact that IF and LDF DR Regimens effect insulin and glucose levels, they effect serum IGF-1 levels (expanded with IF however diminished with LDF) and serum beta-hydroxybutyrate levels (expanded with IF yet diminished with LDF). Diminished IGF-1 levels have been proposed to add to the defensive impact of DR against carcinogenesis. Nonetheless, IF likewise secures against tumor development, proposing that extra instruments should be employable in this valuable impact of IF. Quite compelling concerning the cytoprotective impact of IF was the huge expansion in the degrees of beta-hydroxybutyrate, a fat-inferred fuel utilized when the starch supply is restricting. It is notable that usage of these powers expansions in the fasting state in different tissues including the cerebrum. Since subject on the IF routine gauge significantly more than subject on the LDF routine they may have bigger fat stores and a more prominent ketogenic reaction than that of LDF subject. This shift to ketogenesis may assume an immediate part in the cytoprotective impacts of IF, on the grounds that it has been accounted for that subjects took care of a ketogenic diet show expanded protection from seizures, and that beta-hydroxybutyrate secures neurons in subjects of Alzheimer's and Parkinson's sicknesses. Ketogenic slims down are endorsed for certain patients with epilepsy and are additionally executed in a few mainstream health improvement plans. The discoveries of this investigation recommend that IF can upgrade wellbeing and cell protection from infection regardless of whether the fasting time frame is trailed by a time of gorging with the end goal that generally speaking caloric admission isn't diminished.

The capacity of both the IF and LDF ideal models to improve pressure opposition and expand life range gives a valuable instrument to knowing the system by which DR applies its impact. In the event that a change, for example, an adjusted chemical level is proposed to assume a basic unthinking part, it ought to happen in light of both taking care of systems. Correlation of the two ideal models in this manner gives freedoms to knowing the systems hidden the regulation of maturing rate by DR.

3.4 Intermittent Fasting for the Treatment of Obesity in Adults Aged 18 Years and over

Are intermittent fasting mediations a powerful treatment for overweight and corpulence in grown-ups, when contrasted with regular consideration treatment (ceaseless day by day energy limitation - diminished calorie diet) or no treatment (not indispensable eating routine)?

Background

Overweight and stoutness (delegated Body Mass Index [BMI] of more noteworthy than or equivalent to 25 and 30 individually) is a worldwide general wellbeing worry, with more than 1.9 billion grown-ups overall being overweight in 2014 (more than 600 million of whom are hefty), and bringing about a larger number of passing than underweight. A brought BMI up in adulthood is related with an expanded danger of building up various persistent illnesses which incorporate diabetes, cardiovascular infection, solid skeletal issues and a few malignant growths. Notwithstanding this considerable effect on singular wellbeing and prosperity, there are additionally critical more extensive expenses, for instance, in England the yearly immediate expense for the National Health Service for treating overweight, weight and related bleakness is assessed at over £5 billion pounds, with expenses for the more extensive economy assessed at £27 billion. In this manner successful weight the board is fundamental.

As overweight and heftiness results from a gathering of abundance muscle to fat ratio emerging from an energy lopsidedness - devouring more energy (kcal) than is exhausted - most of weight the executives approaches revolve around practices to address this awkwardness, for example lessening energy consumption through caloric limitation and expanding energy use through actual work. In any case, the etiology of overweight and heftiness is profoundly intricate, including an exchange of natural, mental, cultural and ecological drivers. Thusly, compelling weight the executives is testing, and while there exists a plenty of accessible health improvement plans, not all are exhaustively assessed and thought about, and many weight reduction endeavors bring about weight recover and poor long haul results. It is consequently essentially critical to survey the viability of all new ways to deal with help a proof based way to deal with weight the executives. Intermittent fasting (IF), otherwise called substitute day fasting (ADF), occasional fasting or intermittent energy limitation (IER) is a generally new dietary way to deal with weight the board that includes blending ordinary every day caloric admission with a brief time of extreme calorie limitation/fasting. As far as the conceivable hidden natural advantages of intermittent fasting, there is some proof, overwhelmingly from creature contemplates, to show valuable consequences for weight reduction and cardio-metabolic danger factors. While the supporting robotic proof is restricted, there is some proof to propose that the advantages might be clarified robotically through fat usage and healthful pressure. Anyway current National Institute for Health and Care Excellence (NICE) direction on the treatment of grown-up stoutness doesn't suggest the standard utilization of extremely low calorie counts calories (VLCD) (characterized as a hypo caloric eating regimen of 800 or less kcal/day) for the treatment of grown-up weight. The National Institute for Health and Care Excellence expresses that this methodology ought to possibly be suggested if there is a clinical reasoning for quick weight reduction and should be healthfully finished, part of a multi-segment weight the executive's procedure, including progressing support, and ought to be attempted for a limit of 12 weeks (followed persistently or intermittently). Besides, the British Dietetic Association raises worries that quick weight reduction related with fasting may generally be because of loss of water and glycogen as opposed to fat, and may bring about exhaustion, wooziness and low energy levels. Basically IF includes the intermittent utilization of a VLCD, and there remain inquiries regarding the results of this methodology, regardless of whether there is an ideal fasting example or calorie breaking point, and how economical it is for long haul weight the executives. Intermittent fasting has as of late acquired a lot of ubiquity following critical media consideration. In the UK this dietary methodology arrived at standard after a BBC Horizon narrative broadcasted in August 2012, highlighted an IF approach called the 5:2 eating regimen, which includes five days of ordinary eating designs exchanged with two days of fasting (max 500kcal for ladies and 600kcal for men). Anyway other IF designs are utilized, for example, substitute day fasting. Regardless of the new prevalence of intermittent fasting and related weight reduction guarantees, the supporting proof base in people stays little and there is just one distributed precise survey looking at the medical advantages of this methodology. Anyway the point of this audit was to analyze the effect of this mediation on more extensive medical advantages (not explicitly as a therapy approach for overweight and corpulence), and didn't give an exhaustive system or meta-examination of RCT information. This proposed audit will subsequently address these holes in the proof base.

Review Purpose

Intermittent fasting has been proposed as a potential sustenance approach against heftiness and metabolic illness. In spite of the fact that information from concentrates in subjects convincingly support the antiobesity and cardio metabolic advantages of intermittent fasting, its belongings in human wellbeing are as yet easily proven wrong.

Recent Discoveries

Late examinations have analyzed the impact of two intermittent fasting draws near, that is, substitute day fasting (ADF) and time-limited eating (TRE), on weight reduction and cardio metabolic danger factors. ADF is by all accounts a similarly successful weight reduction way to deal with caloric limitation, however adherence to ADF is really difficult. ADF improves cardio metabolic danger factors, though it might have better metabolic advantages contrasted than caloric limitation in individuals and insulin obstruction. TRE with not obligatory food admission is very much endured and incites 2-4% weight reduction in roughly 3 months. Also, TRE may have metabolic advantages especially in individuals with metabolically strange heftiness even without weight reduction.

Summary

Intermittent fasting is a promising dietary methodology against corpulence and its connected metabolic illnesses. Further examination is expected to: a) set up the drawn out adequacy of TRE in weight reduction and metabolic wellbeing, b) improve the drawn out adherence to ADF and explore its weight reduction free impacts in metabolic wellbeing, and c) decide the instruments fundamental the potential cardio metabolic advantages of intermittent fasting in people.

Insulin opposition is at present a significant medical issue. This might be a direct result of a checked reduction in every day active work during ongoing many years joined with steady food wealth. This way of life slams into our genome, which was in all probability chose in the late Paleolithic time (50,000-10,000 BC) by models that supported endurance in a climate portrayed by variances between times of blowout and starvation. The hypothesis of frugal qualities expresses that these variances are needed for ideal metabolic capacity. We imitated the variances in eight sound youngsters; weight record: 25 kg by exposing them to intermittent fasting each second day for 20 h for 15 days. Euglycemic hyperinsulinemic clips were performed when the mediation period. Subjects kept up body weight. Plasma free unsaturated fat and beta-hydroxybutyrate focuses were, separately, after overnight quick yet expanded (P is equivalent to 0.05) following 20-hours fasting, affirming that the subjects were fasting. Insulin-interceded entire body glucose take-up rates expanded from (P is equivalent to 0.03), and insulin-initiated restraint of fat tissue lipolysis was more unmistakable after than before the mediation (P is equivalent to 0.05). After the 20-hours fasting periods, plasma adiponectin was expanded contrasted and the basal levels when the intercession (P is equivalent to 0.02). This investigation is the first in quite a while to show that intermittent fasting expands insulin-interceded glucose take-up rates, and the discoveries are viable with the frugal quality idea.

To confirm the relationship of intermittent fasting in the bodyweight of overweight and hefty people through a deliberate writing audit. This is an orderly survey dependent on randomized controlled preliminaries. The articles were counseled in the data sets. This survey was assessed through the PRISMA suggestion. : After the choice interaction, four articles were remembered for this survey, looking at intermittent fasting (IF) with calorie limitation diet (CRD) as a benchmark group. In 2 investigations utilizing comparative conventions, there was no critical decrease in body weight of overweight or corpulent subjects. In the other two examinations utilizing various conventions, weight reduction was huge in the IF bunch contrasted with the CRD bunch. Results didn't give proof of the impact of intermittent fasting on weight reduction in overweight or hefty people.

Intermittent fasting, otherwise called intermittent energy limitation, is an umbrella term for different feast timing plans that cycle between intentional fasting (or diminished calorie consumption) and non-fasting over a given period. Strategies for intermittent fasting incorporate substitute day fasting (ADF), intermittent fasting, and day by day time-confined taking care of. A kind of occasional fasting known as the 5:2 eating regimen was promoted in the UK and Australia by Michael Mosley around 2012.

Intermittent fasting may have comparable impacts to a calorie-limitation diet, and has been concentrated in the 21st century as a training to potentially diminish the danger of diet-related infections, like metabolic disorder. A 2019 audit reasoned that intermittent fasting may assist with stoutness, insulin obstruction, dyslipidemia, hypertension, and aggravation.

Intermittent fasting has been censured as a prevailing fashion. The science concerning intermittent fasting is challenged. The American Heart Association expressed in 2017 that intermittent fasting may deliver weight reduction, decrease insulin obstruction, and lower the danger of cardio metabolic infections, in spite of the fact that it is drawn out supportability is obscure. The US National Institute on Aging expressed in 2018 that there is inadequate proof to suggest intermittent fasting, and urges addressing one's medical services supplier about the advantages and dangers prior to rolling out any huge improvements to one's eating design.

There is restricted proof that intermittent fasting produces weight reduction equivalent to a calorie limited eating regimen. Most examinations on intermittent fasting in people have noticed weight reduction, going from 2.5% to 9.9%. Substitute day fasting doesn't influence slender weight, albeit one audit tracked down a little diminishing. Substitute day fasting improves cardiovascular and metabolic biomarkers likewise to a calorie limitation diet in individuals who are overweight, stout or have a metabolic condition.

A recent report which followed an example of 88 hefty ladies more than 10 weeks showed that the individuals who utilized both calorie-limitation and intermittent fasting were more effective at shedding pounds than the gathering who utilized just calorie limitation, or just intermittent fasting. A 2020 investigation of time-confined eating over a three-month term in corpulent individuals, utilizing an example of 116 members, appeared there were no consequences for body weight or metabolic biomarkers, with specialists demonstrating that the examination was too short in length to show an impact on weight reduction.

Intermittent fasting has not yet been concentrated in youngsters, older, or underweight individuals, and might be destructive in these populaces. Intermittent fasting isn't suggested for individuals who are not overweight, and the drawn out supportability of intermittent fasting is obscure starting at 2018.

Conclusion

Typical weight subjects can conform to a 1 feast/day eating routine. At the point when feast recurrence is diminished without a decrease in by and large calorie admission, unobtrusive changes happen in body creation, some cardiovascular illness hazard factors, and hematologic factors. Diurnal varieties may influence results. Subjects who finished the investigation kept up their body weight inside 2 kg of their underlying load all through the 6-month period. There were no huge impacts of supper recurrence on pulse, internal heat level, or a large portion of the blood factors estimated. Be that as it may, while burning-through 1 feast/day, subjects had a huge expansion in hunger; a critical adjustment of body piece, remembering decreases for fat mass; huge expansions in pulse and altogether, LDL-, and HDL-cholesterol focuses; and a huge abatement in convergences of cortisol.

Lightning Source UK Ltd.
Milton Keynes UK
UKHW020642270521
384471UK00010B/730